Code of Ethics and Professional Conduct

College of Occupational Therapists

Revised edition 2015

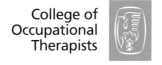

College of
Occupational
Therapists

This edition published in 2015
by the College of Occupational Therapists Ltd
106–114 Borough High Street
London SE1 1LB
www.cot.org.uk

This edition supersedes all previous editions

Author: College of Occupational Therapists
Writer: Henny Pearmain
Category: Standards and strategy

Other enquiries about this document should be addressed to the Professional
Practice Department at the above address.

British Library Cataloguing in Publication Data
A catalogue record for this book is available from the British Library.

While every effort has been made to ensure accuracy, the College of
Occupational Therapists shall not be liable for any loss or damage either directly
or indirectly resulting from the use of this publication.

ISBN 978-1-905944-50-7

Typeset by Servis Filmsetting Ltd, Stockport, Cheshire
Printed in Great Britain by the Lavenham Press, Suffolk

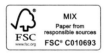

Contents

Preface

i. The *Code of ethics and professional conduct* (hereafter referred to as 'the Code') is produced by the College of Occupational Therapists, for and on behalf of the British Association of Occupational Therapists (BAOT), the national professional body and trade union for occupational therapists throughout the United Kingdom (UK). The College of Occupational Therapists (COT or College) is the subsidiary organisation, with delegated responsibility for the promotion of good practice.

ii. The College is committed to person-centred practice and the involvement of the service user as a partner in all stages of the therapeutic process.

iii. The completion, revision and updating of the Code is the delegated responsibility of the Professional Practice Department of the College. It is revised every five years.

iv. Under the *Health Act 1999* (Great Britain. Parliament) the title 'occupational therapist' is protected by law and can only be used by persons who are registered as such with the regulatory body, the Health and Care Professions Council (HCPC). This means that they will have successfully completed an approved course leading to a diploma or degree in occupational therapy and must be meeting the current HCPC standards and requirements for continued registration. All occupational therapists practising in the UK must be registered with the HCPC.

v. Membership of the British Association of Occupational Therapists is voluntary. It is not a requirement for practice and, although it cannot be a criterion for employment, it provides benefits to support ethical and safe working practice (Great Britain. Parliament 1992). Members of BAOT sign up to abide by this Code, but its content will be relevant and useful to all occupational therapy personnel across the United Kingdom, whether they be members of BAOT or not. It is a public document, so also available to service users and their carers, other professions and employing organisations.

vi. The term 'occupational therapy personnel' includes occupational therapists, occupational therapy students and support workers. It is also pertinent to occupational therapists who are managers, educators and researchers. At times this document also uses the term 'practitioner' in reference to the same range of people.

vii. Where occupational therapy personnel are working in less clearly defined occupational therapy roles or more diverse roles, this code will still apply and should be used to ensure ethical and safe working practice.

viii. This Code should be used in conjunction with the current versions of the HCPC's standards and guidance, along with the College of Occupational Therapists' current professional standards for occupational therapy practice, and local policy.

ix. This Code does not identify every piece of relevant legislation, recognising that some may differ across the four UK nations. Occupational therapy personnel must be aware of and comply with any current European, UK or national legislation and policies, best practice standards, and employers' policies and procedures that are relevant to their area of practice. The relevant areas of legislation are listed in Appendix 1.

This version of the Code supersedes all previous editions (June 2015).

Key terms

Assessment	*A process of collecting and interpreting information about people's functions and environments, using observation, testing and measurement, in order to inform decision-making and to monitor change.*
	(Consensus definition from European Network of Occupational Therapy in Higher Education (ENOTHE) 2004)
Autonomy	*The freedom to make choices based on consideration of internal and external circumstances and to act on those choices.*
	(Consensus definition from ENOTHE 2004)
Best interests	As well as recognising the use of best interests decisions under the *Mental Capacity Act 2005* (Great Britain. Parliament 2005), the approach is extended within the Code to all service users.
	The best interests approach asks whether any proposed course of action is the best one for the patient all things considered.
	(UK Clinic Ethics Network n.d.)

Candour	*Candour is the quality of being open and honest.* (Department of Health 2014, p29)
Capacity (lacking)	For the purpose of the *Mental Capacity Act 2005*: *a person lacks capacity in relation to a matter if at the material time he is unable to make a decision for himself in relation to the matter because of an impairment of, or a disturbance in the functioning of, the mind or brain.* *It does not matter whether the impairment or disturbance is permanent or temporary.* (Great Britain. Parliament 2005, part 1, section 2)
Carer	Someone who provides (or intends to provide), paid or unpaid, a substantial amount of care on a regular basis for someone of any age who is unwell, or who, for whatever reason, cannot care for themselves independently. (Adapted from Great Britain. Parliament 1995) This is sometimes divided into formal carers (care workers) who are paid to give care, and informal carers (often family) who are not paid to provide care.

Competency	*Competence is the acquisition of knowledge, skills and abilities at a level of expertise sufficient to be able to perform in an appropriate work setting.*
	(Harvey 2014)
Continuing professional development (CPD)	*A range of learning activities through which health professionals maintain and develop throughout their career to ensure that they retain their capacity to practise safely, effectively and legally within their evolving scope of practice.*
	(Health and Care Professions Council 2012, p1)
Cost effectiveness	The extent to which an intervention can be regarded as providing value for money.
	(Adapted from Phillips and Thompson 2009)
Delegate	To give an assignment to another person, or to assign a task to another person, to carry out on one's behalf, while maintaining control and responsibility.
Duty of care	A responsibility to act in a way which ensures that injury, loss or damage will not be carelessly or intentionally inflicted upon the individual or body to whom/which the duty is owed, as a result of the performance of those actions.

	A duty of care arises:
	When there is a sufficiently close relationship between two parties (e.g. two individuals, or an individual and an organisation). Such a relationship exists between a service user and the member of occupational therapy personnel to whom s/he has been referred, while the episode of care is ongoing.
	Where it is foreseeable that the actions of one party may cause harm to the other.
	Where it is fair, just and reasonable in all the circumstances to impose such a duty.
	(See Caparo Industries Plc v Dickman 1990)
Ethics	A code of behaviour for personal or professional practice.
Governance	[The systems by which] *organisations are accountable for continuously improving the quality of their services and safeguarding high standards of care.*
	(Adapted from Department of Health 1998, chapter 3)

Handover	To give away or entrust the total care and responsibility for an individual to another. The handover action is complete when the receiving person acknowledges and accepts control and responsibility. This is not to be confused with the role of occupational therapy personnel in a ward handover, where he or she may report information to ward staff, but still retains responsibility for the occupational therapy provided to the service user.
Informed consent	Informed consent is an ongoing agreement by a person to receive treatment, undergo procedures or participate in research, after risks, benefits and alternatives have been adequately explained to them. Informed consent is a continuing requirement. Therefore, occupational therapy personnel must ensure that service users continue to understand the information with which they have been provided, and any changes to that information, thereby continuing to consent to the intervention or research in which they are participating.
	In order for informed consent to be considered valid, the service user must have the capacity to give consent and the consent must be given voluntarily and be free from undue influence.

Must	Where there is an overriding principle or duty.
Occupation	*A group of activities that has personal and sociocultural meaning, is named within a culture and supports participation in society. Occupations can be categorised as self-care, productivity and/or leisure.* (Consensus definition from ENOTHE 2004)
Occupational alienation	*A sense that one's occupations are meaningless and unfulfilling, typically associated with feelings of powerlessness to alter the situation.* (Hagedorn 2001, cited in ENOTHE 2004)
Occupation-centred	*A professional stance to advance 'occupation as the centre of occupational therapy research, education and practice'.* (Nielson 1998, cited in Fisher 2013)
Occupational deprivation	*A state of prolonged preclusion from engagement in occupations of necessity or meaning due to factors outside the control of an individual, such as through geographic isolation, incarceration or disability.* (Christiansen and Townsend 2004, cited in ENOTHE 2004)

Occupational science	*Academic discipline of the social sciences aimed at producing a body of knowledge on occupation through theory generation, and systematic, disciplined methods of inquiry.*
	(Crepeau et al 2003, cited in ENOTHE 2004)
Occupational therapy personnel	For the purpose of this document, this term includes occupational therapists, occupational therapists working in generic or diverse roles, occupational therapy students and support workers working with or for occupational therapists. It is also pertinent to occupational therapists who are managers, educators and researchers.
Practice placement educator	The occupational therapist who supervises students while they are on a practice placement.
Reasonable	An objective standard. Something (e.g. an act or decision) is reasonable if the act or decision is one which a well-informed observer would also do or make.
Service	Within the context of this document the term 'service' usually refers to the occupational therapy service you provide as an individual or group, rather than referring to the occupational therapy department or facility.

Service user	In this Code the term 'service user' refers to any person in direct receipt of any services/interventions provided by a member of occupational therapy personnel in all sectors and all settings.
Should	Where the principle or duty may not apply in all circumstances, in contrast with a 'must' obligation. You should have a justifiable reason for not meeting this requirement.
Sustainable	*Sustainable health care combines three key factors: quality patient care, fiscally responsible budgeting and minimizing environmental impact.* (Jameton and McGuire 2002)

Section One: Introduction

Defining occupational therapy, its values and beliefs

1.1 Occupational therapy has a unique approach to service users. Its beliefs and values have been drawn together and incorporated into the *College of Occupational Therapists' learning and development standards for pre-registration education* (College of Occupational Therapists 2014b).

> *Occupational therapists view people as occupational beings. As occupational beings, people are intrinsically active and creative, needing to engage in a balanced range of activities in their daily lives in order to sustain health and wellbeing. People shape, and are shaped by, their experiences and interactions with their environments. They create identity, purpose and meaning through what they do and have the capacity to transform themselves through conscious and autonomous action.*

> *The purpose of occupational therapy is to enable people to fulfil, or to work towards fulfilling, their potential as occupational beings. Occupational therapists promote activity, quality of life and the realisation of potential in people who are experiencing occupational disruption, deprivation, imbalance or isolation. We believe that activity can be an effective medium for*

remediation, facilitating adaptation and re-creating identity.

(COT 2014b, p2)

The statement on occupational therapy from the World Federation of Occupational Therapists (WFOT) states:

Occupational therapy is a client-centred health profession concerned with promoting health and well being through occupation. The primary goal of occupational therapy is to enable people to participate in the activities of everyday life. Occupational therapists achieve this outcome by working with people and communities to enhance their ability to engage in the occupations they want to, need to, or are expected to do, or by modifying the occupation or the environment to better support their occupational engagement.

(WFOT 2010)

A shorter definition was adopted by BAOT/COT Council in 2004 and published by WFOT in their *Definitions of occupational therapy from member organisations*:

Occupational therapy enables people to achieve health, well being and life satisfaction through participation in occupation.

(WFOT 2013, p48)

The purpose of the Code

1.2 To be deemed as 'competent' you need to demonstrate a combination of knowledge, skills, and behaviours. You may learn knowledge and skills through professional training and/or experience and continuing professional development, but these elements alone are not necessarily what make you a good or safe practitioner. You must also demonstrate behaviours that promote and protect the wellbeing of service users and their carers, the wider public, and the reputation of your employers and your profession. This *Code of ethics and professional conduct* describes a set of professional behaviours and values that the British Association of Occupational Therapists expects its members to abide by, and believe all occupational therapy personnel should follow.

1.2.1 The Health and Care Professions Council (HCPC) has overall responsibility for ensuring that all relevant health professionals meet certain given standards in order to be registered to practise in the United Kingdom. If a formal complaint is made about an occupational therapist, the HCPC will take into account whether their standards have been met. You must know and abide by the requirements of the HCPC.

1.2.2 You have a responsibility to act in a professional and ethical manner at all times. The Code provides a set of values and behaviours that are relevant to you, irrespective of where you work or your level of experience. These values and ensuing attitudes, behaviours and capabilities support and enable professionalism in occupational therapy practice. The Code, along with the College of Occupational Therapists' current professional standards for occupational therapy practice and the HCPC's standards, provide you with a framework for promoting and maintaining good, safe and ethical professional behaviour and practice in occupational therapy.

1.2.3 You should be familiar with the content of the Code. As a practical document, you need to understand its content and how to apply it in your workplace. It should be the first point of reference for you if you have a dilemma related to professional or ethical conduct. Local policy and/or standards should also be adhered to.

1.2.4 Higher education institutions will use the Code throughout students' education to inform them of the required standards of ethics and conduct that occupational therapy personnel are expected to uphold during their academic and professional lives, emphasising its application from point of entry to the programme to the end of their professional career. Higher education institutions are required to ensure that the Code is observed in order to maintain their pre-registration occupational therapy programme's accredited status.

1.2.5 The Code may also be used by others outside the profession to determine the measure of ethical and professional conduct expected of you. The College encourages recognition of the Code by other individuals, organisations and institutions who are involved with the profession, including employers and commissioners.

1.2.6   The Code is a broad document and cannot provide detailed answers to all the specific professional or ethical dilemmas that you might face in your work. If there is uncertainty or dispute as to the interpretation or application of the Code, advice should be sought from the College of Occupational Therapists' Professional Practice Enquiry Service, which may seek an expert opinion if considered necessary.

Section Two: Service provision

Focusing on occupation

2.1 Your practice should be focused on enabling individuals, groups and communities 'to change aspects of their person, the occupation, or the environment, or some combination of these to enhance occupational participation'.

(Adapted from World Federation of Occupational Therapists 2010)

2.1.1 Access to occupational therapy should be based on the occupational needs of the individual, group or community.

2.1.2 Assessment, interventions, outcomes and documentation should be centred on occupational performance, engagement and participation in life roles.

2.1.3 The professional rationale for your intervention or activity should be the enhancement of health and wellbeing through the promotion of occupational performance and engagement.

2.1.4 In this way service users should be empowered to maintain their own health and wellbeing wherever possible.

The occupational therapy process

2.2 You must have and abide by clearly documented procedures and criteria for your service/s.

2.2.1 You should be aware of the standards and requirements of the professional body and the regulatory body, abiding by them as required by registration and/or membership.

2.2.2 You should work in partnership with the service user and their carer/s throughout the care process, respecting their choices and wishes and acting in the service user's best interests at all times.

2.2.3 Following receipt of a referral for occupational therapy, the legal responsibility and liability for any assessment and possible intervention provided by occupational therapy lies with the occupational therapy service to which the case is allocated (see section 3.1.1).

2.2.4 You have the right to refuse to provide any intervention that you believe would be harmful to a service user, or that would not be clinically justified, even if requested by another professional. The guidance given by the Court of Appeal in the case of *R (Burke) v. General Medical Council (Official Solicitor and others intervening)* (2005), is that if a form of treatment is not clinically indicated, a practitioner is under no legal obligation to provide it, although s/he should seek a second opinion. Similarly, a doctor who is responsible for a service user may instruct a therapist not to carry out certain forms of treatment if s/he believes them to be harmful to the service user (Department of Health 1977).

2.2.5   You should maintain an awareness of current policy, guidelines, research and best available evidence, and should incorporate this into your work where appropriate.

2.2.6   A service user can decide not to follow all or part of your recommendations, seeking intervention, equipment or advice elsewhere. This must be recorded in the care record, together with your assessment that the service user has the capacity to make such a decision (see points 3.3.4 and 3.3.5). Provided that you have referred the service user to another agency if appropriate, complied with all the necessary procedures, taken reasonable action to ensure the service user's safety, and ensured that a follow-up is not reasonably required, you will have no further responsibility or liability.

Equality

2.3   You must care for all service users in a fair and just manner, always acting in accordance with human rights, legislation and in the service user's best interests.

2.3.1   You must offer equal access to services without bias or prejudice on the basis of age, gender, race, nationality, colour, faith, sexual orientation, level of ability or position in society. Practice should at all times be based upon the occupational needs and choices of the service user.

2.3.2 You should be aware of and sensitive to how the above factors affect service users' cultural and lifestyle choices, incorporating this into any service planning, individual assessment and/or intervention where possible.

2.3.3 Where possible, the need, or a reasonable request, to be treated, seen or visited by a practitioner with specific characteristics should be met; for example, by a professional and not a student, by a male or female practitioner, or by a particular language speaker.

2.3.4 You must report in writing to your employing authority, at the earliest date in your employment, any religious and/or cultural beliefs that would influence how you carry out your duties. You should explore ways in which you can avoid placing an unreasonable burden on colleagues because of this. This does not affect your duties, as set out in sections 2.3.1 and 2.3.2, and you must always provide service users with full, unbiased information.

2.3.5 It is important to recognise the significance of spiritual, religious and cultural beliefs. If a service user or colleague asks for support, you must ensure that you follow local policy and obtain consent before you seek to meet their spiritual needs. You can offer to find alternative support if you don't feel comfortable in this situation. You must not impose your own faith or belief system onto any situation or person at work.

Resources and sustainability

2.4 Your service and your practice should be centred on the occupational needs of the service user and their carer/s, but local, national and environmental resources for care are not infinite. At times, priorities will have to be identified and choices will have to be made, while complying with legal requirements, and national and/or local policy.

2.4.1 In establishing priorities and providing services, service user and carer choice should be taken into account, and implemented wherever reasonably possible. If the service user lacks the mental capacity to identify his or her preferences, occupational therapy personnel must act in the service user's best interests.

2.4.2 You should work as cost-effectively and efficiently as possible in order to sustain resources. Practitioners are encouraged 'to re-evaluate practice models and expand clinical reasoning about occupational performance to include sustainable practice' (WFOT 2012); for example, considering the health and wellbeing co-benefits of a low carbon lifestyle (Sustainable Development Unit 2014).

2.4.3 You have a duty to report and provide evidence on resource and service deficiencies that may endanger the health and safety of service users and carers to the relevant manager, who should then take appropriate action (Great Britain. Parliament 1998a, section 43B, point (1)d). Local policy should be followed.

2.4.4 Where the service user's or their carer's choice cannot be met, you should explain this to the service user/carer. If you cannot offer, or they will not accept, an alternative, you may provide information as to different service providers, sources of funding, etc. Provided that you have referred the service user to another agency, if appropriate; complied with all the necessary procedures; taken reasonable action to ensure the service user's safety and ensured that a follow up is not reasonably required, you will have no further responsibility or liability.

Risk management

2.5 Risk management is an intrinsic part of governance and the provision of a quality service. Risk management is a process of identifying and adequately reducing the likelihood and impact of any kind of incident occurring that might cause harm. The principles remain the same whether the potential harm is to people, organisations or the environment. The process also enables positive risks to be taken with service users in a safe and appropriate way.

2.5.1 You must familiarise yourself with the risk management legislation that is relevant to your practice, and with your own local risk management procedures.

2.5.2   You are responsible for assessing and managing the identified risks involved in providing care to your service users.

2.5.3   Where care for the service user is shared with or transferred to another practitioner or service, you must co-operate with them to ensure the health, safety and welfare of service users (Great Britain. Parliament 2014 Section 12 (2)(i)).

2.5.4   You are expected to co-operate with your employers in meeting the requirements of legislation and local policy. You must also take reasonable care for your own health and safety and that of others who may be affected by what you do, or do not do (Great Britain. Parliament 1974, section 7).

2.5.5   You must ensure that you remain up to date in all your statutory training related to risk management, health and safety, and moving and handling.

More information is available from the College of Occupational Therapists' current guidance on risk management.

Record keeping

2.6   Record keeping is core to the provision of good quality and safe care. The key purpose of records is to facilitate the care and support of a service user. It is essential to provide and maintain a written or electronic record of all that has been done for/with or in relation to a service user, including any risk assessment and the clinical reasoning behind the care planning and provision. Your records also demonstrate how you meet your duty of care and that your practice is appropriate.

2.6.1   You must accurately and legibly record all information related to your involvement with the service user, as soon as practically possible after the activity, in line with the standards of the Health and Care Professions Council, the College of Occupational Therapists and local policy. Any record must be clearly dated, timed and attributable to the person making the entry.

2.6.2   You must ensure that you meet any legal requirements regarding appropriate data sharing and data confidentiality in record keeping (see section 3.4).

More information is available from the current College of Occupational Therapists' professional standards for occupational therapy practice and guidance on record keeping.

Section Three: Service user welfare and autonomy

Duty of care

3.1 A duty of care arises where there is a sufficiently close relationship between two parties, as with a member of occupational therapy personnel and a service user, and where it is reasonably foreseeable that the actions of one party could, if carelessly performed, cause harm or loss to the other party. Discharging the duty of care requires you to perform your occupational duties to the standard of a reasonably skilled and careful practitioner.

3.1.1 Fulfilling your duty of care

In practice, a duty of care arises when a referral has been received by an occupational therapy service or practitioner. The duty of care would require you to assess the suitability of the potential service user for occupational therapy with reasonable care and skill, following usual and approved occupational therapy practice.

If, as a result of the initial assessment, the individual is not suitable for the receipt of occupational therapy services, then no further duty of care arises other than to inform the referrer of the decision that has been made.

3.1.2 You are required to ensure that all reasonable steps are taken to ensure the health, safety and welfare of any person involved in any activity for which you are responsible. This might be a service user, a carer, another member of staff or a member of the public (Great Britain. Parliament 1974).

3.1.3 Your duty of care would not necessarily stop at the point when a person is discharged from your service or chooses to discharge themselves. Only when you have referred the service user to another agency, if appropriate; complied with all the necessary procedures; taken reasonable action to ensure the service user's safety; and ensured that a follow up is not reasonably required, then you will have no further responsibility or liability.

3.1.4 Breach of duty of care

You may be in breach of your duties to take care if it can be shown that you have failed to perform your professional duties to the standard expected of a reasonably skilled occupational therapy practitioner.

3.1.5 Defences

If it is claimed that you have, in the performance of your duties, breached your duty of care to a service user, it is a good defence to show that a responsible body of like practitioners would have acted in the same way - the Bolam Principle. The Bolam Principle will only be a good defence, however, if it can be shown that the body of opinion relied on has a logical basis and is respectable, responsible and reasonable in its own right. This is the Bolitho Principle (Bolitho v City and Hackney Health Authority 1998).

Welfare

3.2 You must always recognise the human rights of service users and act in their best interests.

3.2.1 You should enable individuals to preserve their individuality, self-respect, dignity, privacy, autonomy and integrity.

3.2.2 You must not engage in, or support, any behaviour that causes any unnecessary mental or physical distress. Such behaviour includes neglect and indifference to pain.

3.2.3 You must protect and safeguard the interests of vulnerable people in your care or with whom you have contact in the course of your professional duties. Vulnerable people should be treated with dignity and respect as equal members of society, entitled to enjoy the same rights and privileges as any one of us would expect. Your duty of care extends to raising concerns, with your manager or an appropriate alternative person, about any service user or carer who may be at risk in any way. Local policy should be followed.

3.2.4 You must always provide adequate information to a service user in order for them to provide informed consent. Every effort should be made to ensure that the service user understands the nature, purpose and likely effect of the intervention before it is undertaken (see section 3.3 on informed consent and mental capacity). This is particularly relevant where there is any element of risk, or where any intervention may cause pain or distress.

3.2.5 You must make every effort not to leave a service user in pain or distress following intervention. Professional judgement and experience should be used to assess the level of pain, distress or risk and appropriate action should be taken if necessary. Advice should be sought when required.

3.2.6 You must support service users and carers if they want to raise a concern or a complaint about the care or service they have received. You should communicate honestly, openly and in a professional manner, receiving feedback and addressing concerns co-operatively should they arise. Advice should be sought when required and local policy followed.

3.2.7 You have a professional duty of candour. You must be open and honest with service users when you become aware that something has gone wrong or someone has suffered harm as a result of your actions or omissions. You should immediately take steps to put matters right and apologise to service users and carers if appropriate to do so.

You must inform your manager/employer and follow local policy.

You must not knowingly obstruct another practitioner in the performance of their duty of candour. You must not provide information, or make dishonest statements about an incident, with the intent to mislead.

3.2.8 If you witness, or have reason to believe, that a service user has been the victim of mistreatment, abuse or neglect in your workplace, you must raise your concerns with your line manager or other prescribed person in order to maintain service user safety.

3.2.9 Everyone has a responsibility to safeguard children, young people and adults at risk. Should you witness, or have reason to believe, that a service user has been the victim of dangerous, abusive, discriminatory or exploitative behaviour or neglect in any setting, you must notify a line manager or other prescribed person, seeking the service user's consent where possible, and using local procedures where available.

3.2.10 If you are an employer or supplier of personnel, you must report to the relevant national disclosure and barring service any person who has been removed from work because of their behaviour, where that behaviour may meet any of the criteria for the individual to be barred from working with children or adults at risk.

3.2.11 You must take appropriate precautions to protect service users, their carers and families, and yourself from infection in relation to personal, equipment and environmental cleanliness. Local infection control guidance and policy should be followed.

Informed consent and mental capacity

3.3 You have a continuing duty to respect and uphold the autonomy of service users, encouraging and enabling choice and partnership working in the occupational therapy process.

Informed consent is an ongoing agreement by a person to receive treatment, undergo procedures or participate in research after risks, benefits and alternatives have been adequately explained to them. Informed consent is a continuing requirement. Unless restricted by mental health and/or mental capacity legislation, it is the overriding right of any individual to decide for himself (herself) whether or not to accept intervention.

A service user can only give informed consent if he or she has the mental capacity to do so. A mentally incapacitated service user cannot validly consent to or refuse treatment, nor can his relatives/carers consent on his behalf.

3.3.1 Where service users have mental capacity, they have a right to make informed choices and decisions about their future and the care and intervention that they receive. Where possible, such choices should be respected, even when in conflict with professional opinion.

3.3.2 Service users with capacity should be given sufficient information, in an appropriate manner, to enable them to give consent to any proposed intervention/s concerning them. They should be able to understand the nature and purpose of the proposed intervention/s, including any possible risks involved.

3.3.3 For consent to be valid, it must be given voluntarily by an appropriately informed person who has the capacity to consent to the intervention in question. The giving of consent, whether verbal or written, must be recorded.

3.3.4 You should, as far as possible, support people in making their own choices. Where a service user's capacity to give informed consent is restricted or absent, you should try to ascertain and respect their preferences and wishes, at all times seeking to act in their best interests. All decisions and actions taken must be documented. You must attempt to provide alternative ways for a service user to give or withhold consent if speech is not possible.

3.3.5 You must assess service users' mental capacity to make decisions in relation to occupational therapy provision, in accordance with current legislation. If the service user does not have capacity, you must consider whether the proposed treatment is in the service user's best interests, having regard to the factors and consultation requirements of the legislation

Code of ethics and professional conduct

and codes of practice, before commencing treatment.

3.3.6   Most service users have the right to refuse any intervention at any time in the occupational therapy process. This must be respected and recorded in the care record. You must not coerce or put undue pressure on a service user to accept intervention, but must inform them of any possible risk or consequence of refusing treatment. For service users without capacity, a 'best interests' decision is required.

3.3.7   Practitioners should be aware of current legislation, codes of practice and relevant guidance in relation to mental capacity and consent.

Further advice is available from the Department of Health; the Department of Health, Social Services and Public Safety for Northern Ireland; the Scottish Executive; and the Welsh Assembly Government.

Confidentiality

3.4   You are obliged to safeguard confidential information relating to service users at all times. It is established law that confidential personal information must be protected and a failure to do so can lead to a fine, or give the service user a cause of action for breach of confidence. The same rights and restrictions apply to material stored or transferred electronically and when communicating with others via any medium, including virtual/online communities and networks.

3.4.1 You must make yourself aware of your legal responsibilities under the *Data Protection Act 1998,* the *Human Rights Act 1998* (Great Britain. Parliament 1998b, 1998c) and mental health/capacity legislation.

3.4.2 You must keep all records, in any format, securely, making them available only to those who have a legitimate right or need to see them.

3.4.3 The disclosure of confidential information regarding the service user's diagnosis, treatment, prognosis or future requirements is only possible where: the service user gives consent (expressed or implied); there is legal justification (by statute or court order); or it is considered to be in the public interest in order to prevent serious harm, injury or damage to the service user or to any other person. Local procedures should be followed.

3.4.4 For the purposes of direct care, relevant personal confidential data should be shared among registered and regulated health and social care professionals who have a legitimate relationship with the service user, following guidance on implied consent (DH 2013, p14).

3.4.5 You must adhere to local and national policies regarding confidentiality in the storage, movement and transfer of information at all times, including via electronic/digital means.

3.4.6 You must grant service users access to their own records in accordance with relevant legislation. Reference should be made to current guidance/policy (both local and national) on access to personal health and social care information.

3.4.7 You must obtain and record consent prior to using visual, oral, written or electronic/digital material relating to service users outside of their care situation, e.g. for learning/teaching purposes. Service user confidentiality and choice must be observed in this circumstance.

3.4.8 Discussions with or concerning a service user should be held in a location and manner appropriate to the protection of the service user's right to confidentiality and privacy.

See also section 6.1.8 in relation to confidentiality in research.

More information on confidentiality is available from the current version of the College of Occupational Therapists' guidance on record keeping.

Section Four: Professionalism

Professional conduct

4.1 As practitioners you are not just accountable for your competence, but also for your actions and behaviours, both inside and external to the workplace.

4.1.1 You must be aware of and take responsibility for the impression and impact you make on others, conducting and presenting yourself in a professional manner while in your work role.

4.1.2 You must be aware of and take responsibility for your conduct outside of your work role, in situations where your behaviour and actions may be witnessed by your colleagues, your employer, your service users and/or the public.

4.1.3 You must be aware of and take responsibility for your conduct when using any form of social media. See section 4.1.2. The content of this Code should be applied to social media use, whether for work or personal purposes.

4.1.4 You should adhere to statutory and local policies at all times.

Professional and personal integrity

4.2 You must act with honesty and integrity at all times. You must not engage in any criminal or otherwise unlawful or unprofessional behaviour or activity which is likely to damage the public's confidence in you or your profession.

4.2.1 You must not undertake any professional activities when under the influence of alcohol, drugs or other intoxicating substances.

4.2.2 You must not promote and/or use illegal substances in the workplace.

4.2.3 You must inform your employers and the regulatory body if you are convicted of a criminal offence, receive a conditional discharge for an offence, or if you accept a police caution.

4.2.4 You must inform the regulatory body if you have had any restriction placed upon your practice, been suspended or dismissed by an employer, or similar organisation, because of concerns about your conduct or competence.

4.2.5 You should co-operate with any investigation or formal enquiry into your own professional conduct, the conduct of another worker or the treatment of a service user, where appropriate.

The professionalism of colleagues

4.3 Any reference to the quality of work, or the integrity of a professional colleague should be expressed with due care to protect the reputation of that person. Any concern must be objective, evidence-based where possible and raised through appropriate channels.

4.3.1 Should you have reasonable grounds to believe that the behaviour or professional performance of a colleague may be deficient in standards of professional competence, you should notify the line manager or other appropriate person in strictest confidence. This includes (but is not limited to) when a colleague's performance is seriously deficient, when he or she has a health problem which is impairing his or her competence to practise, or when he or she is practising in a manner which places service users or colleagues at risk.

4.3.2 If you become aware that something has gone wrong or someone has suffered harm as a result of your colleagues' actions or omissions, you should raise your concerns with a line manager or other appropriate person and follow local policy.

4.3.3 If you become aware of any intentional malpractice, criminal conduct or unprofessional activity, whether by occupational therapy personnel or other staff, you should raise your concerns with a line manager or other appropriate person and follow local policy.

4.3.4   In reporting any concerns to a line manager or other appropriate person, the information must be objective, relevant and limited to the matter of concern.

4.3.5   If you are aware of discrimination, bullying and harassment in the workplace, you must adhere to statutory and local policies with regard to reporting it.

4.3.6   You may give evidence in court concerning any alleged negligence of a colleague. Such evidence must be objective and capable of substantiation.

4.3.7   When providing a second opinion to a service user and/or their carer, it must be confined to the case in question and not extend to the general competence of the first practitioner.

Personal profit or gain

4.4   You should not accept tokens such as favours, gifts or hospitality from service users, their families or commercial organisations when this might be construed as seeking to obtain preferential treatment (Great Britain. Parliament 1889, 1906, 1916). In respect of private practice this principle still prevails in terms of personal gain.

4.4.1   Local policy should always be observed in the case of gifts.

4.4.2   If a service user or their family makes a bequest to a practitioner or a service, this should be declared according to local guidelines.

4.4.3   You must put the interests of the service user first and should not let this duty be influenced by any commercial or other interest that conflicts with this duty; for example, in arrangements with commercial providers that may influence contracting for the provision of equipment.

Information and representation

4.5   Information and/or advertising, in respect of professional activities or work, must be accurate. It should not be misleading, unfair or sensational.

4.5.1   You should accurately represent your qualifications, education, experience, training, competence and the services you provide. Explicit claims should not be made in respect of superiority of personal skills, equipment or facilities.

4.5.2   You should not claim another person's work or achievements as your own unless the claim can be fully justified. You should respect the intellectual property rights of others at all times.

4.5.3   You may only advertise, promote or recommend a product or service in an accurate and objective way. You may not support or make unjustifiable statements about a product or service.

4.5.4 If you are aware that possible misrepresentation of the protected title 'occupational therapist' has occurred, you must contact the Health and Care Professions Council.

Relationships with service users

4.6 You should foster appropriate therapeutic relationships with your service users in a transparent, ethical and impartial way, centred on the needs and choices of the service user and their family/carers.

4.6.1 It is unethical for you to enter into relationships that would impair your judgement and objectivity and/or which would give rise to the advantageous or disadvantageous treatment of a service user.

4.6.2 You must not enter into relationships that exploit service users sexually, physically, emotionally, financially, socially or in any other manner.

4.6.3 You must not exploit any professional relationship for any form of personal gain or benefit.

4.6.4 You should avoid entering into a close personal relationship with a current service user. You are responsible for maintaining an appropriate professional relationship. If there is a risk that the professional boundary may be broken, this should be disclosed and discussed with your manager. You should hand over therapy care for the service user to an appropriate professional colleague.

4.6.5 In the case of relationships, sexual or otherwise, regardless of when the professional relationship may have started or ended, or however consensual it may have been, it will always be your responsibility to prove that you have not exploited the vulnerability of the service user and/or his or her carer, should concerns be raised.

4.6.6 As far as is reasonably practical, you should not enter into a professional relationship with someone with whom you already have, or have had, a close personal relationship. This includes family members and friends. Where there is no reasonable alternative you must make every effort to remain professional and objective while working with the individual you know or have known. In such circumstances this should be disclosed and discussed with the service manager and a note should be made in care records. This is for your protection as much as for the service user.

Fitness to practise

4.7 You must inform your employer/appropriate authority and the Health and Care Professions Council about any health or personal conditions that may affect your ability to perform your job competently and safely.

4.7.1 You should limit or stop working if your performance or judgement is affected by your health.

More information on informing the regulatory body is available from *Guidance on health and character* (HCPC 2014).

Section Five: Professional competence and lifelong learning

Professional competence

5.1 You must only provide services and use techniques for which you are qualified by education, training and/or experience. These must be within your professional competence, appropriate to the needs of the service user and relate to your terms of employment.

> 5.1.1 You should achieve and continuously maintain high standards in your professional knowledge, skills and behaviour.

> 5.1.2 You should be aware of and abide by the current legislation, guidance and standards that are relevant to your practice, remaining up to date with relevant training where necessary.

> 5.1.3 You should understand the scope and benefits of emerging information and communication technologies to ensure that you can make best use of what is available in your own practice, or through referral to other agencies.

> 5.1.4 If you are asked to act up or cover for an absent colleague, or if you are asked to take

on additional tasks, such duties should only be undertaken after discussion, considering additional planning, support, supervision and/or training.

5.1.5   Adequate training and support should be provided to enable you to be competent to carry out any additional tasks or responsibilities asked of you.

5.1.6   You should be given the opportunity to raise any concerns and be provided with the rationale behind the original request. If you find that you cannot agree to such a request you should contact your local union representative for advice and support.

5.1.7   If you are seeking to work in areas with which you are unfamiliar or in which your experience has not been recent, or if you take on a more diverse role, you must ensure that you have adequate skills and knowledge for safe and competent practice and that you have access to appropriate support.

Delegation

5.2   If you delegate interventions or other procedures you should be satisfied that the person to whom you are delegating is competent to carry them out. In these circumstances, you, as the delegating practitioner, retain responsibility for the occupational therapy care provided to the service user.

5.2.1 You should provide appropriate supervision for the individual to whom you have delegated the responsibility.

Continuing professional development

5.3 You must undertake continuing professional development (CPD) through a range of learning activities to ensure that your practice is safe, legal and effective, according to the requirements of the Health and Care Professions Council. You must maintain a continuous, up-to-date and accurate record of your CPD activities (HCPC 2012, p6).

See the College of Occupational Therapists' *Code of continuing professional development* (COT 2014a) in Appendix 1.

5.3.1 Employing organisations and managers are encouraged to recognise the value of continuing professional development to individual practitioners, the service and service users.

5.3.2 You should be supported in your practice and development through regular professional supervision, whether provided locally or via long-arm support.

5.3.3 If you have expert or high-level knowledge, skills and experience, you have a responsibility to share these with your colleagues through supervision, mentoring, preceptorship and teaching opportunities.

More information is available from the *Joint position statement on continuing professional development for health and social care practitioners* (Royal College of Nursing et al 2007), the current version of the COT supervision guidance and HCPC guidance on supervision.

Collaborative working

5.4 You should respect the responsibilities, practices and roles of other people with whom you work.

5.4.1 You should be able to articulate the purpose of occupational therapy and the reason for any intervention being undertaken, so promoting the understanding of the profession.

5.4.2 You should recognise the need for multiprofessional and multiagency collaboration to ensure that well co-ordinated services are delivered in the most effective way.

5.4.3 You have a duty to refer the care of a service user to another appropriate colleague if it becomes clear that the task is beyond your scope of practice. You should consult with other service providers when additional knowledge, expertise and support are required.

5.4.4 If you and another practitioner are involved in the treatment of the same service user, you should work co-operatively, liaising with each other and agreeing areas of responsibility. This should be communicated to the service user and all relevant parties. Consent must be sought before sharing information.

Occupational therapy practice education

5.5 You have a professional responsibility to provide regular practice education opportunities for occupational therapy students where possible, and to promote a learning culture within the workplace.

5.5.1 You should recognise the need for individual education and training to fulfil the role of the practice placement educator and, where possible, undertake programmes of study.

5.5.2 If you undertake the role of practice placement educator, you should provide a learning experience for students that complies with the *College of Occupational Therapists' learning and development standards for pre-registration education* (COT 2014b) and current professional standards, and is compatible with the stage of the student's education or training.

5.5.3 If you accept a student for practice education, you should have a clear understanding of the role and responsibilities of the student, the educational institution and the practice educator.

More information is available from the *College of occupational therapists' learning and development standards for pre-registration education* (COT 2014b).

Section Six: Developing and using the profession's evidence base

6.1 As research consumers, you must be aware of the value and importance of research as the basis of the profession's evidence base.

    6.1.1   You should be able to access, understand and critically evaluate research and its outcomes, incorporating it into your practice where appropriate.

    6.1.2   You should evaluate the effectiveness and efficiency of the services that you provide, and undertake audits against appropriate available standards.

    6.1.3   You should incorporate evidence-based outcome measures into your practice and research activity to demonstrate effectiveness of intervention and services.

    6.1.4   When undertaking any form of research activity, you must understand the principles of ethical research and adhere to national and local research governance requirements.

6.1.5   When undertaking any form of research activity, you should abide by national, professional and local ethics approval and permission processes.

6.1.6   When undertaking any form of research activity, you must protect the interests of service users, fellow researchers and others.

6.1.7   When undertaking any form of research activity you must establish and follow appropriate procedures for obtaining informed consent, including regard to the needs and capacity of participants.

6.1.8   When undertaking any form of research activity, you must protect the confidentiality of participants throughout and after the research process.

6.1.9   You should disseminate the findings of your research activity through appropriate publication methods in order to benefit the profession and service users, and to contribute to the body of evidence that supports occupational therapy service delivery.

Appendix 1: Legislation

You are expected to be familiar and comply with any current European, UK or national legislation and policies, best practice standards, and employers' policies and procedures that are relevant to your area of practice. The *Code of ethics and professional conduct* does not identify every piece of relevant legislation, recognising that many differ across the four UK nations. Areas of legislation and guidance that are relevant to this document include:

Candour

Clinical governance

Confidentiality – data protection and sharing, access to records/freedom of information

Consent

Equality

Health and safety/safe working practice

Health and social care

Human rights

Mental health and mental capacity

Record keeping

Reporting and disclosure

Risk assessment and management

Safeguarding

Sexual offending

Appendix 2: College of Occupational Therapists code of continuing professional development

The purpose

The College of Occupational Therapists (COT) has devised this *Code of continuing professional development* (COT 2014a) to support the occupational therapy workforce by setting out clear expectations for all BAOT (British Association of Occupational Therapists) members' professional development.

It is aligned with, and complementary to, Health and Care Professions Council (HCPC) requirements for registrants, and does not replace the regulatory requirements of HCPC for professional development and adherence to their standards for continuing professional development (HCPC 2012).

This code places responsibility upon all occupational therapy personnel to extend their professional development beyond regulatory requirements in order to ensure a fulfilling career journey that sustains the profession in changing contexts and provides the best outcomes for service users.

This code should be interpreted by individual members to reflect their specific practice environment and level of expertise.

The code of continuing professional development

i. You are personally responsible for ensuring that you continue to learn, develop and enhance your professional skills and practice abilities as an occupational therapy professional and embed them in your practice.

ii. Development activities will ensure that, at a minimum, you are able to practise in a safe and reliable manner, centred around your service user/s and their occupational engagement.

iii. Your critical reflective thinking and development will take account of:

    a. Your personal values beliefs and attitudes.
    b. Your professional capability.
    c. Your practice context.
    d. Relevant current and future policy.

iv. Learning and development opportunities occur in both professional and personal areas of life and may be formal or informal. These experiences can support and evidence professional development if considered through a critically reflective approach and applied to occupational therapy practice. You will be able to demonstrate how you turn every suitable experience into a learning opportunity.

v. Critical reflective thinking underpins the bringing together of different ideas and application of all professional development activities to the benefit of your service user/s, your service and yourself. You will be able to demonstrate how you have developed your critically reflective thinking skills throughout your professional journey.

vi. You will undertake systematic formal reflection; for example, through annual appraisal and regular supervision, on your:

    a. Current professional skills and practice abilities as an occupational therapy professional.

    b. Current context of practice and service needs.

    c. Personal beliefs and values as they relate to your professional life.

This appraisal (or systematic formal reflection) will be informed, where possible, by service user and colleague feedback and should form the baseline for your professional development strategy and plan.

vii. You will establish, maintain and actively pursue a professional development strategy that considers your current role, supports your future career path and gives direction to your learning. A plan to fulfil this strategy will be identified to ensure all the development opportunities that you undertake have purpose and meaning to you.

viii. As applicable to your professional role you will be able to demonstrate how your professional development plan positively impacts on:

    a. The experience of service users.

    b. The quality of services provided now and in the future.

    c. Your professional identity as an occupational therapy practitioner.

ix. Your professional development activities will work to support organisational needs and be shared with relevant others, including fellow occupational therapists, associate members and other professionals.

References

Bolitho v City and Hackney Health Authority [1998] AC 232 (HL).

R (Burke) v. General Medical Council (Official Solicitor and others intervening) [2005] EWCA Civ 1003, [2006] QB 273. Available at: *http://www.familylawweek. co.uk/site.aspx?i=ed409* (paragraph 50) Accessed on 12.01.15.

Caparo Industries Plc v Dickman [1990] 2 AC 605 (HL).

Christiansen CH, Townsend EA (2004) *Introduction to occupation: the art and science of living*. Upper Saddle River, NJ: Prentice Hall.

College of Occupational Therapists (2014a) *Code of continuing professional development*. London: COT.

College of Occupational Therapists (2014b) *College of Occupational Therapists' learning and development standards for pre-registration education.* London: COT.

Crepeau EB, Cohn ES, Schell BAB eds (2003) *Willard and Spackman's occupational therapy*. 10th ed. Philadelphia: Lippincott Williams & Wilkins.

Department of Health (2014) *Requirements for registration with the Care Quality Commission: response to consultations on fundamental standards, the Duty of Candour and the fit and proper persons requirement for directors.* London: DH. Available at: *https://www.gov.uk/government/uploads/system/ uploads/attachment_data/file/327561/Consultation_ response.pdf* Accessed on 12.01.15.

References

Department of Health (2013) *Information: to share or not to share: government response to the Caldicott review.* London: DH. Available at: *https://www.gov.uk/government/uploads/system/uploads/attachment_data/file/251750/9731-2901141-TSO-Caldicott-Government_Response_ACCESSIBLE.PDF*
Accessed on 12.01.15.

Department of Health (1998) *A first class service: quality in the new NHS.* London: DH. Available at: *http://webarchive.nationalarchives.gov.uk/+/www.dh.gov.uk/en/publicationsandstatistics/publications/publicationspolicyandguidance/dh_4006902*
Accessed on 27.01.15.

Department of Health (1977) *Relationships between medical and remedial professions.* (HC (77) 33). London: DH.

European Network of Occupational Therapy in Higher Education Terminology Project Group (2004) *Occupational therapy terminology database.* Amsterdam: ENOTHE. Available at: *http://pedit.hio.no/~brian/enothe/terminology/* Accessed on 12.01.15.

Fisher A (2013) Occupation-centred, occupation-based, occupation-focused: same, same or different? *Scandinavian Journal of Occupational Therapy, 20(3),* 162–173.

Great Britain. Parliament (2014) *Health and Social Care Act 2008 (Regulated Activities) Regulations 2014.* (SI 2936). London: Stationery Office. Available at: *http://www.legislation.gov.uk/ukdsi/2014/9780111117613/contents* Accessed on 12.01.15.

Great Britain. Parliament (2005) *Mental Capacity Act 2005.* London: Stationery Office. Available at: *http://www.legislation.gov.uk/ukpga/2005/9/contents*
Accessed on 13.01.15.

Code of ethics and professional conduct

Great Britain. Parliament (1999) *Health Act 1999.* London: Stationery Office. Available at: *http://www. legislation.gov.uk/ukpga/1999/8/contents*
                                    Accessed on 13.01.15.

Great Britain. Parliament (1998a) *Public Interest Disclosure Act 1998.* London: Stationery Office. Available at: *http://www.legislation.gov.uk/ ukpga/1998/23/contents*   Accessed on 13.01.15.

Great Britain. Parliament (1998b) *Data Protection Act 1998.* London: Stationery Office. Available at: *http:// www.legislation.gov.uk/ukpga/1998/29/contents*
                                    Accessed on 13.01.15.

Great Britain. Parliament (1998c) *Human Rights Act 1998.* London: Stationery Office. Available at: *http:// www.legislation.gov.uk/ukpga/1998/42/contents*
                                    Accessed on 13.01.15.

Great Britain. Parliament (1995) *Carers (Recognition and Services) Act 1995.* London: HMSO. Available at: *http://www.legislation.gov.uk/ukpga/1995/12/contents*
                                    Accessed on 13.01.15.

Great Britain. Parliament (1992) *Trade Union and Labour Relations (Consolidation) Act 1992.* London: HMSO. Available at: *http://www.legislation.gov.uk/ ukpga/1992/52/contents*   Accessed on 13.01.15.

Great Britain. Parliament (1974) *Health and Safety at Work Act 1974.* London. HMSO. Available at: *http:// www.legislation.gov.uk/ukpga/1974/37*
                                    Accessed on 13.01.15.

Great Britain. Parliament (1889, 1906, 1916) *Prevention of Corruption Acts 1889 to 1916.* London: HMSO.

Hagedorn R (2001) *Foundations for practice in occupational therapy.* 3rd ed. Edinburgh: Churchill Livingstone.

Harvey L (2014) *Analytic quality glossary.* [s.l]: Quality Research International. Available at: *http://www. qualityresearchinternational.com/glossary/ competence.htm*   Accessed on 27.01.15.

Health and Care Professions Council (2014) *Guidance on health and character.* London: HCPC. Available at: *http://www.hpc-uk.org/publications/*
                                        Accessed on 12.01.15.

Health and Care Professions Council (2012) *Continuing professional development and your registration.* London: HCPC. Available at: *http://www. hpc-uk.org/publications/*   Accessed on 12.01.15.

Jameton A, McGuire C (2002) Toward sustainable health-care services: principles, challenges, and a process. *International Journal of Sustainability in Higher Education, 3(2),* 113–127.

Neilson C (1998) The issue is how can academic culture move towards occupation-centered education? *American Journal of Occupational Therapy, 52(5),* 386–387.

Phillips C, Thompson G (2009) *What is cost effectiveness?* 2nd ed. London: Hayward Medical Communications.

Royal College of Nursing, Institute of Biomedical Science, Unison, British Academy of Audiology, Royal College of Midwives, British Association of Art Therapists . . . Chartered Society of Physiotherapy (2007) *A joint statement on continuing professional development for health and social care practitioners.* London: RCN.

Sustainable Development Unit (2014) *Sustainable, resilient, healthy people & places: a sustainable development strategy for the NHS, public health and social care system.* Cambridge: SDU. Available at: *http://www.sduhealth.org.uk/documents/ publications/2014%20strategy%20and%20 modulesNewFolder/Strategy_FINAL_Jan2014.pdf*
Accessed on 08.03.15.

UK Clinic Ethics Network (undated) *Mental Capacity Act: determining best interests.* (Educational Resources). Available at: *http://www.ukcen.net/index. php/education_resources/mental_capacity/ determining_best_interests*   Accessed on 25.01.15.

World Federation of Occupational Therapists (2013) *Definitions of occupational therapy from member organisations.* Forrestfield, AU: WFOT. (This document can be accessed from the Resource Centre, filter resources by category: 'General'). Available at: *http:// www.wfot.org/resourcecentre.aspx*
Accessed on 14.01.15.

World Federation of Occupational Therapists (2012) *Environmental sustainability, sustainable practice within occupational therapy.* (Position Statement). Forrestfield, AU: WFOT. (Position statements can be accessed from the Resource Centre, filter resources by category: 'Position Statements'). Available at: *http:// www.wfot.org/resourcecentre.aspx*
Accessed on 14.01.15.

World Federation of Occupational Therapists (2010) *Statement on occupational therapy.* Forrestfield, AU: WFOT. (Position statements can be accessed from the Resource Centre, filter resources by category: 'Position Statements'). Available at: *http://www.wfot.org/ resourcecentre.aspx*   Accessed on 14.01.15.

Bibliography

For the most recent versions of College of Occupational Therapists' publications please visit www.cot.org.uk/publications

College of Occupational Therapists (2015) *Supervision.* London: COT.

College of Occupational Therapists (2011) *Professional standards for occupational therapy practice.* London: COT. Available at: *http://www.cot.co.uk/standards-ethics/professional-standards-occupational-therapy-practice*   Accessed on 12.01.15.

College of Occupational Therapists (2010) *Risk management.* 2nd ed. London: COT.

College of Occupational Therapists (2010) *Record keeping.* 2nd ed. London: COT.

College of Occupational Therapists (2010) *Code of ethics and professional conduct.* London: COT.

Department for Constitutional Affairs (2007) *Mental Capacity Act 2005 code of practice.* London: Stationery Office. Available at: *https://www.gov.uk/government/uploads/system/uploads/attachment_data/file/224660/Mental_Capacity_Act_code_of_practice.pdf*   Accessed on 12.01.15.

Department of Health (2009) *Reference guide to consent for examination or treatment.* 2nd ed. London: DH.

Great Britain. Parliament (2006) *Safeguarding Vulnerable Groups Act 2006*. London: Stationery Office. Available at: *http://www.legislation.gov.uk/ukpga/2006/47/contents*　　Accessed on 14.01.15.

Great Britain. Parliament (2000) *Freedom of Information Act 2000.* London: Stationery Office. Available at: *http://www.legislation.gov.uk/ukpga/2000/36/contents*　　Accessed on 13.01.15.

Great Britain. Parliament (1983) *Mental Health Act 1983*. London: HMSO. Available at: *http://www.legislation.gov.uk/ukpga/1983/20/contents*　　Accessed on 14.01.15.

Health and Care Professions Council (2013) *Standards of proficiency: occupational therapists*. London: HCPC. Available at: *http://www.hpc-uk.org/publications/*　　Accessed on 12.01.15.

Health and Care Professions Council (2012) *Standards of conduct, performance and ethics*. London: HCPC. Available at: *http://www.hpc-uk.org/publications/*　　Accessed on 12.01.15.

Health and Care Professions Council (2012) *Your guide to our standards of continuing professional development*. London: HCPC. Available at: *http://www.hpc-uk.org/publications/*　　Accessed on 12.01.15.

Health and Care Professions Council (2010) *Guidance on conduct and ethics for students*. London: HCPC. Available at: *http://www.hpc-uk.org/publications/*　　Accessed on 12.01.15.

Royal College of Nursing (2011) *Spirituality in nursing care: a pocket guide*. London: RCN. Available at: *http://www.rcn.org.uk/__data/assets/pdf_file/0008/372995/003887.pdf*　　Accessed on 02.02.15.

World Federation of Occupational Therapists (2005) *Code of ethics*. Forrestfield, AU: WFOT.